How to Survive Peer Review

How to Survive Peer Review

Elizabeth Wager

Publications Consultant, Sideview, Princes Risborough, Buckinghamshire, UK

Fiona Godlee

Editorial Director for Medicine, BioMed Central, London, UK

Tom Jefferson

Director, Health Reviews Ltd, Anguillara Sabazia, Roma, Italy

© BMJ Books 2002
BMJ Books is an imprint of the BMJ Publishing Group

All rights reserved. No part of this publication may be reproduced,
stored in a retrieval system, or transmitted, in any form or by any
means, electronic, mechanical, photocopying, recording and/or
otherwise, without the prior written permission of the publishers.

First published in 2002
Second impression 2003
by BMJ Books, BMA House, Tavistock Square,
London WC1H 9JR

www.bmjbooks.com

British Library Cataloguing in Publication Data

A catalogue record for this book is available from the British Library

ISBN 0 7279 1686 6

Typeset by SIVA Math Setters, Chennai, India
Printed and bound by GraphyCems, Navarra

Contents

1: Introduction

> *Peer*
> *vb intr. 1. to look intently with or as if with difficulty.*
> *2. to appear partially or dimly.*
> *n. 1. a person who is an equal in social standing, rank,*
> *age, etc.*
>
> Collins Dictionary of the English Language,
> London & Glasgow: Collins, 1979.

Peer review is inescapable if you want to get a grant, have your research published in a journal or presented at a conference, or want to develop your academic or clinical career. At some stage in your career, you are also likely to be asked to review an abstract, manuscript or grant proposal and will probably be expected to do this with little guidance, on the basis of having undergone the process yourself.

This book aims to explain just enough about peer review to enable you to survive and benefit from it, and to be a competent reviewer. It is designed to be a practical handbook, based on evidence and experience but not weighed down with footnotes and references. It is the equivalent of a phrase book that enables you to order a beer, get directions to your hotel, and enjoy your holiday without becoming an expert in literature or linguistics.

It does not attempt to debate the merits of peer review, what purpose it serves, how well it meets its aims, or how it could be improved. If you find the subject interesting and want to take it further, you will find other, more academic, books listed in the Further Reading section. Not surprisingly, we particularly recommend another book edited by two of us*, which covers many of these topics in detail.

Although the term "peer review" usually relates to the important milestones of funding and publication, the concept of critical discussion of ideas and findings runs through the entire scientific process. The principles that will help you to survive formal peer review can therefore usefully be applied to many other situations, so we have included a chapter on informal peer review.

If you search the medical literature for the term "peer review" you will discover articles on professional appraisal, especially in relation to nursing. We have therefore included a short chapter to acknowledge this special use of the term. While reviewing an individual's performance is, in many ways, different from reviewing a single piece of work, there are many similarities, and it is interesting to consider how differently other forms of peer review might have evolved if they took place face to face. However, it is beyond the scope of this modest book to provide comprehensive guidelines on performance evaluation and, again, we refer interested readers to other works for more detail.

This book is based both on our experiences of peer review and on many other people's research on the subject, which we acknowledge here rather than in traditional references and footnotes. We particularly thank, for their support and for use of their material, Drummond Rennie, Richard Smith, Trish Groves, Chris Bulstrode, David Moher, Alejandro Jadad, Doug Altman, Ken Schulz, Anna Donald, Dave Sackett, Brian Haynes, Gordon Guyatt, and Peter Tugwell. We also acknowledge the reviewers of this book, Frank Davidoff and Tim Albert, for their helpful and thoughtful comments, and we thank our many colleagues and friends who have contributed to *Peer Review in Health Sciences**, to stimulating debates at the International Congresses on Peer Review, and to the Cochrane reviews on peer review. Finally, we thank A. D. Malcolm who gave us the idea for this book in a review of *Peer Review in Health Sciences*.

A note on how to use this book

Although most people submit work for peer review before they are asked to act as reviewers, learning to think like a reviewer will help you understand the process. So, even though you may be tempted to skip straight to the chapter on surviving peer review, we encourage you to read the two preceding chapters first.

---

* Godlee F, Jefferson T (eds) *Peer review in health sciences*. London: BMJ Books, 1999.

2: What is peer review?

Although the term peer review is familiar to virtually all scientists and clinicians, it is rarely defined and is used to cover a number of different functions often performed by different groups of people. The term is most often used to describe a formal system whereby a piece of academic work is scrutinised by people who were not involved in its creation but are considered knowledgeable about the subject. However, it is also used to describe professional appraisal processes used to assess the performance of an individual, team, or department.

Scientific journals or meetings use peer review to inform the process of selecting items for publication or presentation. Funding bodies use it to decide which projects to support. Journals and some meetings also use the process to improve selected work. The term also encompasses comment and criticism by readers after publication of an article – so-called "post-publication peer review". Thus, peer review acts as both a filter for selection and a quality control mechanism.

Strictly speaking, one would expect peer review to relate only to assessment by members of a peer group, that is colleagues at exactly the same stage of their careers. However, the term is usually applied more broadly to include evaluation by journal editors, editorial boards, selection committees, and senior colleagues. Suggestions for improvement may also come from junior colleagues or professional technical editors. Like most other processes of scientific endeavour, peer review is therefore a collaborative effort, and so we have taken an inclusive approach rather than limit our discussions to strict but artificial definitions of the process or the players.

Journal peer review

Thousands of biomedical journals use some form of peer review to help editors decide what to publish. Journals fall into two groups, based on the underlying philosophy of their selection process. Most use a "top-down" approach. These journals receive many more submissions than they can publish, and use peer review to cream off the most interesting. The long-established, general medical journals, which originated in paper-based production, all use this method. They reject 80–90% of submissions and use peer review to identify those of greatest relevance to their readers and most likely to affect clinical practice. The same system, but with slightly less alarming rejection rates, is used by specialist journals. Again, they use peer review not only to distinguish sound and ethical research, but also to identify the findings most likely to interest their readers.

Electronic publishing, which frees publishers from the distribution costs and space constraints of traditional paper and ink, has fostered an alternative approach. Some electronic journals, while still peer reviewed, operate a bias towards publication. Their philosophy is to accept anything that meets their minimum standards. In other words, they take a "bottom-up" approach. They use peer review to weed out submissions that are incomprehensible or that report research that is ethically or methodologically unsound – but they let readers select the items that interest them by means of electronic searching and alerts. These journals do not expect their readers to be interested in everything that they publish and they make available sound research that may be of interest to only a small audience.

Even before the advent of electronic publishing, a few paper journals adopted the "bottom-up" approach. They overcame the problems of production costs by requiring authors to pay for publication, either directly through page charges or by agreeing to buy reprints. These so called "pay journals" are largely used by pharmaceutical companies, which appreciate short turnaround times and are willing to pay for publication. Such companies are not bothered by the fact that these journals have few subscribers because they can use their own representatives to distribute reprints. The pay journals enable companies to publish results of routine or repeated studies that are required for drug registration but are unlikely to be accepted by major journals. Publishing in a peer reviewed journal gives more credibility than if companies publish studies themselves, and also makes findings permanently accessible via electronic databases.

Table 2.1 Pros and cons of different peer review systems for authors

System	Advantages	Disadvantages
Top-down/ "creaming off"	Prestigious journal Detailed review	High chance of rejection Slow decision-making
Bottom-up/ "weeding out"	High chance of acceptance Rapid decision-making	Less prestigious journal Cost (processing charges/ page charges/reprints)

Beyond this important distinction between top-down and bottom-up selection, most variations in peer review are superficial. However, these minor variations can affect the timing and, to some extent, the output of the process. The use of different systems appears to depend more on a journal's history and resources than on any research that one system is better than another.

Journal peer review systems

Single editor, all externally reviewed

The simplest system of peer review involves a single editor and a pool of reviewers. The editor (usually an academic who performs this role on top of a full-time job) scans all submissions. Apart from articles that are clearly unsuitable for the journal, all submissions are sent out to between one and four reviewers. The editor usually asks reviewers whether they think that the submission should be published, and will expect an answer supported by a detailed review that includes suggestions for improving the submission. If most reviewers recommend publication, the editor will accept their decision. If they disagree, he or she may seek further review. Although the editor has the final say, the reviewers' views on acceptance will be influential and, for this reason, such journals may refer to them as referees since they largely determine the fate of submissions.

If you submit your work to a journal like this you can expect to wait several months for a decision. The editor has a day job to do and few resources with which to chase tardy reviewers. The editor will also wait for all reviews to be completed before making a decision. On the positive side, you can expect to receive two or more detailed critiques of your paper, which may make helpful suggestions for improvements.

If you review for this type of journal you can expect to receive submissions of varying quality, some of which may not be suited to the journal, but you will be expected to provide a detailed review and a recommendation about whether the item should be published.

Editorial board with occasional further review

Another system adopted by journals run by academic societies with unpaid editors is to use an editorial board to review virtually all submissions. The board is selected to provide a range of expertise, and other reviewers will rarely be used. In such journals, the editor scans the submission then sends it to the relevant member(s) of the board. This method may be slow, since board members are expected to review large numbers of papers. You may therefore receive a less detailed review than under the first system.

As a member of an editorial board you must be prepared to review large numbers of papers, covering a relatively broad range of topics.

In-house staff plus external review

Larger, wealthier journals have a full-time professional editor and staff. The in-house editors act like an editorial board. They tend to be generalists with a good understanding of research methodology, the journal's aims, and its readers' interests. They review all submissions and are responsible for rejecting 30–50% without external review. If your paper is rejected after in-house review you will receive a rapid decision (in weeks rather than months) but may not receive a detailed critique. If you are rejected in this way, it usually means that you chose the wrong journal in terms of its scope or prestige. All submissions that the in-house editors regard as potentially publishable are sent to external reviewers. The decision

Table 2.2 What to expect from different peer review systems

Type	Speed of decision	Feedback
In-house	Rapid if rejected at this stage (days or weeks)	Reason for rejection (sometimes short review)
External review	Slow (weeks or months)	Detailed review
Additional review	Even slower	Detailed, multiple reviews

Table 2.3 Examples of journals that use different peer review systems

Method	Journals
External review	*American Journal of Obstetrics and Gynecology* BioMed Central journals
Editorial board	*Circulation*
In-house +/− external review	*Lancet* *JAMA*
In-house +/− external review + expert committee	*BMJ*

Table 2.4 Who does what in different peer review systems?

Journal type	Gives opinion on acceptance	Suggests improvements	Final decision on publication	Copy editing
Large general	In-house editor	In-house editor, External reviewer	Committee/ Editor	Professional technical editor
Academic society	Referee	Referee	Editorial board/Editor	Professional technical editor/ Editorial board
Electronic	Reviewer	Reviewer	Editor	Usually none
Small specialist	Referee	Referee/Editor	Editor	Editor

process is slower than internal review, but you will receive a detailed critique.

If you review for such journals you are less likely to be asked if you recommend publication. This decision usually rests with the in-house editorial team, the editor-in-chief, or an editorial committee. Because all papers have gone through in-house review those sent out to reviewers are likely to be of more uniform quality and more appropriate to the journal than those from journals that send out all submissions. Large journals also tend to have large databases of reviewers, so you can expect to receive papers on a narrow range of topics close to your own research interests.

Additional review

If reviewers disagree about the merits of a submission, or it is highly technical, it may undergo further review. Statistical review is often done after papers have been fully reviewed by content experts. This is because suitably qualified reviewers are rare and journal editors do not want to overburden them. Any additional review is likely to delay decision-making.

Editorial boards and committees

Some journals use an editorial board or committee for the final decision. These groups are usually chaired by the editor-in-chief, meet regularly to discuss the reviewers' comments, and then decide which submissions to accept for publication. This final stage has little effect on the timing of decisions, unless the committee meets infrequently.

How are reviewers chosen?

Most journal editors inherit a database of reviewers listing their areas of expertise. The list expands with the editors' personal contacts and as reviewers are identified from people who submit work to the journal. Reviewers can also be identified from among the authors of articles cited in the submitted manuscript, or from searches of Medline or other electronic databases. Some journals record the performance of reviewers and prune out those who provide superficial or abusive reviews or consistently miss deadlines. Some journals encourage authors to nominate suitable reviewers or to warn against those with conflicting interests. However, the final choice of reviewer rests with the editor.

Requests to review may be passed around departments or delegated to junior staff. Authors have no protection against this and, indeed, research suggests that younger scientists are more diligent and produce better reviews than their superiors. Editors expect to be told if a review request is passed onto a colleague.

Masked and open review

After some studies suggested that reviewers may be prejudiced by an author's identity or place of work, some journals adopted masked (or blinded) review. The aim of masking is to minimise personal biases and make the review process more objective. Masking is performed by removing the authors' details from the submission before review. More recent research shows that it is difficult (and costly) to successfully blind reviewers to an author's identity because of their familiarity with the research community and the tendency among authors to cite their own work. There is also conflicting evidence about whether masked review is, in fact, more objective than unmasked.

Traditionally, the reviewer's identity is not revealed to the author. This, again, is based on the assumption that anonymity will increase objectivity and honesty. Studies have shown that authors often think that they can identify reviewers, but they are usually incorrect. Some journals practise open reviewing, in which the reviewers are asked to sign their reviews and even to have their signed comments posted on the journal's website if the article is accepted. Potential benefits of open reviewing include greater accountability on the part of the reviewers, and credit for the work they have done. A potential weakness of open review is that reviewers may feel inhibited about expressing their true feelings. Even if authors know or guess the reviewer's identity they are usually expected to conduct discussions via the journal and not to contact reviewers directly.

Conflict of interest

Many journal editors ask reviewers to reveal reasons why they might be unable to produce an objective review. This is referred to as declaring a "conflict of interest". The most obvious conflicts are financial ones, such as being paid by, or investing in, companies that sell the medical products or services being studied in the manuscript under review. Personal, political, or ideological conflicts are harder to quantify and detect, and probably less often revealed.

Such conflicts are more likely to come to light if authors know the reviewer's identity. Use of several reviewers should also dilute the effect of a biased reviewer. If you believe that a reviewer has an undeclared conflict of interest you could discuss this with the journal editor. However, since most journals are not prepared to reveal the identity of their reviewers, this may prove difficult.

Copy editing

Once a submission has been accepted, it usually undergoes copy editing, which ensures that it follows the journal's house style and involves further checks on accuracy and consistency. Copy editing may therefore contribute as much as other aspects of peer review designed to improve the quality of the work, although it is often assumed to be less important.

Editors of small, specialist journals sometimes do the copy editing themselves, but, in larger establishments, it is done by professional technical editors. These people are not necessarily experts in the journal's subject matter, but they are experts in preparing papers for publication and are good at picking up errors and inconsistencies. For example, technical editors will spot columns that add up to 101% and references that are incomplete. They may even pick up important errors overlooked by authors and reviewers. They will reword ungrammatical or ambiguous sentences and apply the journal's house style. This governs things like the way terms are abbreviated, spelling preferences (US or UK, -ize or -ise) and heading styles. Paper journals tend to invest more in copy editing than electronic publications.

Peer review of conference abstracts

Many of the principles set out for journal peer review apply to conference abstracts. Scientific meetings usually use a selection committee, which performs a similar function to an editorial board. They may be assisted by external reviewers, or may review all abstracts themselves. Similar to the practice for journal submissions, some conferences remove author details from abstracts before sending them out to reviewers in an attempt to reduce bias and increase objectivity.

The major difference between most meetings and journals is that reviewers are rarely asked to suggest ways of improving abstracts, and authors are rarely given the chance to revise them. The process is therefore simply a filter to decide whether a piece of work is accepted for presentation.

Peer review of grant proposals

This, again, follows similar patterns to journals, usually using several external reviewers to comment on a proposal. However, reviewers almost always know the identity of the applicant, and may even be provided with a full curriculum vitae (resumé) in order to assess whether the researcher is sufficiently qualified and experienced to perform the proposed work.

Other types of peer review

Book proposals

If you approach a publisher with an idea for a book, your outline will probably be shown to one or two advisors before a decision is made. These reviewers may also be asked to read your submitted typescript. Book publishers, like journals, also employ technical editors. The processes described for journals generally apply. The reviewers will almost always be told who the authors are, and the identity of the reviewers may be revealed to the authors.

Peer review within the Cochrane Collaboration

The type of peer review carried out within the Cochrane Collaboration during the preparation of systematic reviews is different from editorial peer review. Cochrane systematic reviews have an agreed format and the full report follows on from an agreed (and published) protocol, which has itself been peer reviewed. The system is designed to minimise the adversarial aspects of other systems. An editorial review group oversees the process, which involves invited reviews from several external experts in the field. Peer review by consumers is encouraged and specific guidelines have been prepared for them (see www.cochrane.org and www.cochraneconsumer.com for more information). The Collaboration also encourages post-publication peer review and expects authors to correct and update their work in the light of comments from readers.

3: How to be a reviewer

Good peer reviewers play a crucial part in the advancement of science and are highly valued by journal editors, conference organisers and funding bodies. As open peer review becomes more widely practised, they are also gaining recognition from authors and other members of the scientific community. But becoming a good reviewer takes time and practice, and finding help or advice on how to review a piece of scientific work can be difficult. This chapter will tell you some of what you need to know.

Rules for reviewing anything

- Read the instructions to find out what you are being asked to do and why.
- If you receive no instructions and are not clear about what you are being invited to do, ask for more information or decline the request.
- Review the work not the person (unless you have been asked to do this), and don't try to be clever.
- Admit your limitations.
- Be as objective as possible and take account of (and declare) any conflicts of interests.

How to review journal articles

Being invited to review

The invitation to review may come by email, fax, post, or telephone. Some journals give only the title of the paper, while others send out the full paper and instructions on how to proceed. It is flattering to be invited, especially if the journal is well known. But before agreeing to review the manuscript, ask yourself the following questions.

- *Is the manuscript within my field of expertise?* If you haven't been given enough information to decide this, ask for more. Ideally the manuscript will be on a subject that you are currently working on, since this means that you will be well up on the current literature. If you are not sure whether you know enough about the content or methods described in the article to produce a good review, say no to the invitation.

- *Am I happy with the journal's peer review process?* Some journals now have open peer review, which means that the author will be told who the reviewers are. Some also now ask reviewers to allow their signed comments to be posted on a website if the manuscript is accepted. Open review increases accountability and gives reviewers credit for the work they do. If you are not comfortable with open review, this is your chance to decline. Similarly, if you have strong feelings against anonymous review, or some other aspect of the peer review process, now is your chance to express them.

- *Do I have time to do this review?* Surveys of reviewers suggest that most reviewers take between two and five hours to complete a review, but if you are doing it for the first time, you should put aside between eight and twelve hours. Some reviews can take as long as 48 hours. Later on we'll describe what is involved in producing a proper peer review report, which may explain why it can take so long.

- *Can I meet the deadline?* Most journals ask reviewers to complete a review within 2–3 weeks. Some also have fast-track peer review procedures, which ask for a review within 48 hours. Remember how frustrating it is as an author to wait for a decision on a paper. Only agree to review if you can deliver the report on time.

- *Do I have any conflicts of interest?* These include anything that might unfairly affect your view of the manuscript, either positively or negatively, such as working closely with (or being married to) one of the authors, working in a rival group, working for or having shares in the company that makes the drug being tested, or working for a rival company. Some journals ask reviewers to declare conflicts of interest. If the journal doesn't ask, tell them anyway, and if you're not sure whether you have a conflict of interest or not, contact the editors and ask their advice.

If you decide NOT to accept the invitation to review

- Tell the journal immediately so that the editors can look for alternative reviewers.

- Suggest alternative reviewers if you can. Finding the right reviewers is one of the most difficult aspects of editorial peer review, so most editors will thank you for this.

If you agree to review

- Let the journal know and confirm the deadline. Ask for any additional information. If you are not familiar with the journal, ask the editorial office to send you a copy, and a copy of the instructions to authors.
- The journal is likely to provide you with some forms to complete, and some instructions for reviewers. Read these before embarking on your review.
- Having agreed to review the manuscript, do everything you can to submit your report on time. If circumstances change and you are unable to review the paper on time, let the journal know as soon as possible.
- Keep it confidential. While under review, the manuscript is a confidential document. Don't discuss it with others without prior permission from the journal. After reviewing the manuscript, return it to the journal or destroy it. Don't keep copies.
- Don't contact the authors except with the journal's permission. Even journals that have an open reviewing policy may prefer to keep the reviewers' identities hidden until a decision on the manuscript has been reached. Most journals like to mediate between reviewers and authors rather than have them discussing things among themselves.
- Do as you would be done by. Aim to be as objective, constructive, conscientious, and systematic as possible. These attributes separate the best reviewers from the rest.

Assessing the manuscript

Three questions to ask of every research report

- *Do I understand it?* Are the question and the methods clearly explained?
- *Do I believe it?* Are the conclusions justified by the data and are the methods valid?
- *Do I care?* Is the question important and interesting?

While reading the manuscript through, ask yourself the following questions.

- *Is the research question or objective clearly stated?* Is it clear from the manuscript why the authors did the study? Do the authors summarise and reference the existing literature adequately and accurately?
- *Is the research question interesting and important?* Remember that the question matters more than the answer. This means that if the question has been clearly stated and is important, the answer is important whatever it is (positive, negative, or neutral).
- *Is the work original?* To check this, you may need to do a literature search. The term "original" means different things in different contexts, but in its broadest sense it includes the reporting of new data, ideas, or methods, or the reanalysis of existing data. If the question has been addressed before, does this manuscript add enough new information to justify publication? If you think the research is not original, give references to previous work: don't just say "It's not original". If you know of important studies that the authors don't refer to, provide the references.
- *Is the work valid?* To answer this question, you must ask several questions. Is the study design right for answering the study's main question? Were the subjects sampled correctly? Were the controls appropriate and adequate? Was a power calculation required and, if so, was it done before the study started? Was there a high enough response rate? Are the methods adequately described? Were the analyses done correctly? Do the numbers add up? For more detailed checklists see p. 51.
- *Are the conclusions supported by the data?* Conclusions overstating the findings are very common and may need to be corrected in the title and the abstract as well as in the main body of the paper.
- *Is the work well presented?* Is the writing clear and coherent? Is the manuscript structured appropriately? Check for the correct balance between text, tables, and figures: the text should tell the story, the tables should provide the detailed data, and the figures should illustrate the story. Are there

any discrepancies between the text, tables, and figures, or between the abstract and the main text? Make a note of important spelling mistakes (ones that the editors may not pick up such as misspelled names), but leave detailed copy editing to the technical editor.

- *Are there any ethical problems?* Does the manuscript mention ethical approval for the study by an ethics committee or institutional review board? Did the authors obtain informed consent? Is there any sign of research misconduct?
- *Is there a fatal flaw?* If you think you have identified a fatal flaw in the work, it makes little sense to do a full review of it. Your review should make clear what the flaw is, including supportive references, and explain why you believe it is irremediable.
- *Should the journal publish the work?* Some journals want reviewers to advise on whether or not to publish. Others want only an objective critique of the paper, to help inform their editorial decision. Either way it is helpful to address the question of whether you think the manuscript should be published at all, and whether you think it fits the journal in question. You may feel that you need to see a revised version before making this decision.
- *Should the journal commission any accompanying commentaries?* If you know the journal and its audience well enough, you may want to alert the editors to a particularly important and relevant piece of work, and suggest names of people (including yourself if appropriate) to write a commentary.

Writing your report

The aim of the report is twofold: to help the editors decide what to do with the paper, and to help the authors improve it before publication.

- Have another look at the journal's instructions for reviewers. Some journals send forms with tick boxes to record each aspect of the manuscript, but there is usually also space for free text comments.
- Head any separate documents with the paper's title and other identifying information.

- Begin with a brief outline of the paper. This shows the authors and editors that you have understood the paper.
- Number your comments. This helps the authors when responding and the editors when judging the author's response. Indicate which comments relate to which parts of the manuscript.
- Don't submit handwritten edits on the margins of the paper. These are hard for journals to pass on to authors.
- Stick to what you know. Don't feel you have to cover all aspects of a paper. Make clear to the editors where your expertise ends so that they will know when to consult additional reviewers.
- Acknowledge help from others. If, after asking the editors, you have shared the task of reviewing the paper with colleagues, acknowledge their help in your report.
- Don't get personal or make disparaging comments. Focus on the paper not the author. Remember that the purpose of review is not to annihilate someone else.
- Be courteous and constructive. An important aim of peer review is to improve manuscripts before they are published. Authors are more likely to accept criticism if the first thing they read is positive. Remember to identify strengths as well as weaknesses.
- Don't allow the best to be the enemy of the good. The study may not be perfect but it may be the best that can be achieved under the circumstances. If the data are important but the study is flawed, it may still be useful to publish the paper. The authors should be asked to acknowledge any weaknesses in their study, and the journal may wish to commission a commentary using the paper to highlight problems as a lesson in research methodology.
- Mention all conflicts of interest. Journals usually ask you to declare only personal and professional ties with the authors and financial interests (such as stocks and shares) that may be affected by publication of the paper. You can also mention other types of conflicting interest, such as strongly held scientific, political, or religious beliefs that might have influenced your judgement.
- Send your report in on time. If you need more time, contact the journal so that they know what's going on and can warn the authors of any delay.

Some frequently asked questions

How do journals handle disagreement between reviewers? Disagreement between reviewers is common, both on specific points within a manuscript and on the question of whether the work should be published. In-house editors employed by larger journals will usually assess each set of comments alongside the manuscript and reach their own decision. Editors of smaller journals who rely on the reviewers to decide on publication will usually resolve the matter by sending the manuscript to a third reviewer.

Will I get any feedback about my review? The journal should let you know its final decision about the paper and show you the comments of the other reviewers. Read these to see if there are important problems with the manuscript that you might have missed, and compare the comprehensiveness and tone of your review with those of your co-reviewers.

Will I be asked to look at the manuscript again? Most journals ask reviewers whether they want to see the manuscript again after it has been revised. This is a key part of responsible reviewing, to see whether the authors have adequately addressed your concerns. If you have raised substantial concerns and criticisms about the submission, you should offer to see it again after revision. The journal should provide a covering letter from the authors outlining the changes that they have made in response to your comments. If the journal does not provide this, ask for it, as it makes the task of re-reviewing substantially easier.

What tools are available to help me with critical appraisal of different study designs? Several validated checklists now exist (see Further reading, p. 49), as well as checklists derived from evidence-based publications (see p. 51). These can help to minimise subjectivity and to ensure that the important aspects of a manuscript are assessed.

How to review conference abstracts

Once you have accepted an invitation to review abstracts for a meeting, make sure that you are clear about what the organisers want of you, and if you are not, contact them. Organisers won't be too impressed if your review comes with a disclaimer that you didn't know exactly what the meeting was about.

The meeting organisers should have weeded out abstracts that don't meet the submission criteria in terms of format, length, and subject matter, so you should be able to concentrate on the content. Meeting organisers have to arrange the review of hundreds of abstracts in a relatively short time, so filtering may be less effective and administrative mistakes more likely than in papers submitted to journals. Before starting your review, it is wise to count the abstracts that you have received and check them against the number specified in the covering letter or email. Next check that the titles, numbers, and content of the abstracts are consistent with what you expected.

Read any instructions that you are sent and check whether you are expected to use a scoring system or checklist. In many cases, reviewers for conferences are asked only whether a piece of work should be accepted or rejected since abstracts are submitted as camera-ready copy and cannot be changed. Check if this is the case but, if not, you may be invited to suggest how the abstracts could be improved. You may also be asked to say whether they would be more suited to oral or poster presentation.

Assessing the abstracts

Many of the questions that you should ask yourself when assessing abstracts are the same as those for assessing work submitted to journals (see above), the main difference being that you have less information to go on. Some abstracts will have been written before the full results of the study are available but, if so, the authors should make this clear. Check with the meeting organiser if this type of "place-holder" abstract is acceptable. You will rarely be in a position to judge whether results will be available in time for the meeting but you should be able to decide whether the research addresses an interesting question and whether the proposed methods are sound.

Despite the space constraints, a good abstract should manage to give the main features of the study question and methods, and make clear the important findings and conclusions. If you cannot understand the abstract, it is likely that nobody else will be able to either, so you should reject it.

Writing your report

Again, similar rules apply as for peer review of journal submissions (see above). Above all, follow the organiser's instructions. Clearly label each set of comments with the title and number of the abstract, and be as constructive as possible.

How to review grant proposals

When reviewing a research proposal, you are, in essence, being asked to decide whether it is likely to reflect a good investment for the funding body and for society in general. This means deciding whether the study is needed, whether the methods proposed are appropriate, and whether the researchers are up to the job.

Assessing the proposal

- *Is the study needed?* Look for a clear justification from the researchers, including a thorough review of the existing literature, preferably in the form of a systematic review. But don't rely on this – do your own additional searches of the literature and if possible a search for similar studies already under way.
- *Are the methods appropriate?* The main difficulty is in distinguishing between the quality of the proposal and the quality of the proposed study. There is little hard evidence that a good proposal makes a good study; but a coherent and comprehensive proposal is a good sign, and a sound method minimises the risks. The questions for assessing journal submissions (see above) and the checklists at the

end of the book (p 51) provide a framework for assessing research methods.

- *Are the researchers up to the job?* The funding body may not expect you to assess this, or to comment on the authors' financial report – this may be for other reviewers. However, if you are asked to assess these things, you will need information about the researchers' track record (from their curricula vitae) and their current resources, and an understanding of the costs of this kind of research. A good research proposal will include a clear project plan, indicating when and why additional staff and other resources will be needed, and giving milestones and process outcomes for judging how the project is progressing. If this is not included, you can request it.

Writing your report

As with journal peer review, make sure you are clear about what is being asked of you, make sure you understand what was required of the researchers when they submitted their proposal, and be as constructive as possible.

If the application for funds is successful, you may be asked to review periodic reports of progress, especially if the investment is substantial.

4: Surviving peer review

Surviving peer review of journal articles

What authors can expect of journal editors and reviewers

Authors are entitled to reviews that are thorough, knowledgeable, timely, and courteous. However these qualities are hard to define and, like common sense, less common than one might hope.

If a reviewer has completely misunderstood your work, or overlooked a crucial feature, you can discuss this with the editor and request another review. If your paper has been rejected after in-house review you could request external review, but this may be a waste of time if the editor is convinced that your work is not suited to the journal.

If you have not had a response for several months, check whether the journal publishes target response times. If you haven't heard within the target period, contact the journal office and ask what is happening.

Editors usually remove stinging criticism or personal invective before reviews are sent to authors. If you receive a discourteous review, you should inform the editor. This may not affect the decision on your article but may alert the journal to avoid this reviewer in future or to tell him or her that such personal attacks are unacceptable.

If the review process is open and you know that the reviewer has failed to declare an important conflict of interest that may have affected the journal's decision, let the editor know.

Step-by-step guide for submitting research to a peer reviewed journal

1 *Choose the right journal.* Spend time considering the implications of your research, your intended audience, and

the message you want to communicate. Ask colleagues which journals they read and respect. Browse back issues to understand the journal's style and scope. Check that the format you have chosen is acceptable (for example, don't send a review article to a journal that only publishes original research or vice versa).

2 *Keep the journal and your intended audience in mind as you write.* Ask yourself, "Why would these people want to read my paper?" Consider the aspects of your findings that would particularly interest them: focus on these and cut down on everything else. Check for specific instructions about the length and format of submissions and stick to these.

3 *Consult the journal's instructions to authors and other useful sources of information.* Ideally, you should identify your journal and check its specific "Instructions to authors" before you start writing. General guidance on topics such as authorship, conflict of interest, and other important aspects of publication can be found in the *Uniform Requirements for Submission to Biomedical Journals* prepared by the International Committee of Medical Journal Editors (available at www.icmje.org).

If your manuscript reports a randomised controlled trial, the CONSORT guidelines provide an excellent checklist, which many journals ask authors to follow. Get the latest version from www.consort-statement.org.

4 *When you've finished writing, read the instructions to authors again.* Few things exasperate editors more than authors who ignore their instructions. Although ground-breaking findings are unlikely to be rejected because of a few typographical errors or references in the wrong style, paying attention to detail usually pays off. For a start, a well-prepared submission puts editors and reviewers in a good mood. Furthermore, a carefully written submission is more likely to instil confidence. A manuscript full of mistakes or which fails to follow instructions does not create an image of a diligent and conscientious researcher. References in the wrong style or a dog-eared copy might suggest that work has been rejected by another journal.

Points to check when you've finished writing

Abstract: Does it fit the journal's maximum length and format (with or without headings)? Does it accurately reflect the manuscript?
Keywords: Check if these are required and, if so, whether they need to conform to NLM MeSH headings.
Title: Is it concise and informative? Do you need to supply a short title (running head) for use on the header of subsequent pages?
Layout: Have you double spaced everything – even tables, figure captions, and references? Have you indicated the text position of tables and figures? Have you included captions for tables and figures?
Acknowledgements: Have you acknowledged the source of funding?
Conflicts of interest: Have you declared all of these? (It is good practice to include a declaration in the manuscript as well as in the covering letter so that reviewers can see this.)
Ethics: Have you mentioned ethics committee (review board) approval?

5 *Start gathering the things you need for the submission package as soon as possible.* By the time you come to submit a paper you will be either fed up with it after umpteen revisions and tedious wranglings with your co-authors or up against a deadline. Either way you will want to submit it as quickly as possible. You will therefore be tempted to shove it in the post without checking everything. This is not the best way to appear intelligent and well organised. Check the items that you will need and have them ready before the final draft stage to avoid last-minute stress.

Items that often cause last-minute panics

- Full names, qualifications and affiliations of all authors
- Full contact details of corresponding author (phone, fax, email, full postal address)
- Authors' signatures and statement of contributorship (describing who did what, which some journals ask for); these can be separate from the covering letter and prepared well in advance
- Copyright form (which may have to be signed by all authors)
- Consent to reproduce copyright material or patients' photographs or medical details

(continued)

- Signed agreement from anyone mentioned in the acknowledgements (sometimes required by American journals)
- Conflict of interest form
- Documentation of "personal communications"
- Evidence of "in press" citations (for example, a copy of the acceptance letter from the journal)

6   *Remember what the reviewers and editors will have to do.* Most journals want everything double spaced with wide margins on numbered pages. This is to help technical editors mark up the copy into the journal's house style and note any queries on the paper. It also makes the paper easier for reviewers to read.

If you are submitting a file on disk there may be other requirements, for example:

- leave the right edge unjustified (ragged);
- use tab commands not spaces when creating tables;
- put all tables and figures at the end of the document (don't paste them into the text).

To facilitate author anonymity, if required by the journal, put author details on a separate title page (start the abstract on the next page). Do not include authors' names in headers, footers or file names.

7   *Write a good covering letter.*

- Use headed paper to indicate where you work.
- Get the editor's name right (check a recent edition of the journal – sending a letter to the previous editor or misspelling the editor's name does not inspire confidence.)
- Get the journal's name right (if the manuscript has been rejected by one journal, make sure you change the journal name on the covering letter when submitting elsewhere.)
- Describe, very briefly, what you found and why this is relevant to readers. Don't just use a neutral description of your research (for example: We are submitting a study to determine the onset of action of Wonderdrug X vs

Patentpill Y); say what you showed (for example: Our study demonstrates that Patentpill Y reduces nausea and vomiting significantly faster than Wonderdrug X).

- Briefly explain the key message and implications of your findings but don't oversell your work or claim that it will change the face of medicine if it won't.
- Tell the editor why you are submitting to that particular journal.
- Show an understanding of the journal's readership and/or previous related publications. If possible, give the editor a reason for publishing your paper (for example, if it complements an earlier piece published by the journal).
- Consult the instructions to authors for necessary wording, for example:

  - this research has not been published before and this paper is not being considered for publication by any other journal;
  - all of the undersigned authors have approved the final version;
  - all authors fulfil the authorship criteria.

8 *Submit your paper.* Do this only after having read the instructions to authors yet again to check that you've included all the bits and pieces.

What happens after you have submitted your paper

Journals usually acknowledge receipt of submissions and may assign a reference number for further correspondence. Once you have received this acknowledgement, all you can do is wait – or perhaps start work on your next paper. A few journals (notably the pay journals and electronic ones) aim to make a decision in a couple of weeks. For all the rest, the decision-making process usually takes from 3–6 months.

A letter (or email) giving details of the decision is sent to the corresponding author. Depending on the system and outcome of the review (see tables in Chapter 2), you will also receive reviewers' comments. It is up to the corresponding author to keep the other authors informed of this. If you are not the corresponding author, you will have no direct contact with the journal.

Four things can happen to your submission:

- outright rejection
- rejection with an invitation to make major changes and resubmit
- acceptance conditional on responding to reviewers' comments
- unconditional acceptance.

What to do if your submission is rejected

If your work is rejected after in-house review, you probably chose the wrong journal. Do some more research about journal readerships and the types of paper that they publish. Alternatively, it may indicate that there is a major flaw in your work, so think about your findings critically, discuss them with colleagues, and be honest about their implications and limitations. If you received reviewers' comments, read them carefully after the initial disappointment has worn off. Put them away for a couple of days, then read them again and decide, with your co-authors, whether to change the paper.

Resubmitting to the same journal is not usually worthwhile. However, if you feel that your paper has been completely misunderstood, or you are able to answer major criticisms, for example by including additional data, it might be worth appealing against a decision in a well-argued letter to the editor. In most cases, however, it is better to swallow your pride and submit somewhere else. Don't be too disheartened – with perseverance most work can be published somewhere!

What to do if you get a conditional acceptance

Very few submissions are accepted unconditionally. Virtually all acceptances are therefore conditional on the authors responding to the reviewers' comments. The important thing to remember is that you do not have to make all the changes that the reviewers suggest, but you do have to answer all their concerns. If you are unwilling to change something you must give convincing reasons for this. If reviewers give conflicting advice, seek guidance from the editor. Don't forget to look at the editor's covering letter, which often includes further requests for changes.

If the revisions seem quite minor, and the co-authors agree, one author may revise the paper but should let the others know what he or she is doing, and send them a copy of the revised version. If major changes are suggested, it may be helpful to meet and discuss them and divide the work between authors.

After you have revised your manuscript, prepare a response describing what you have done. Address each point in order. If reviewers number their comments, use this system for your response. If you have not made a suggested change, give the reasons. Where you have made changes, provide page and paragraph references so that the editor or reviewer can find them easily.

Be polite but not obsequious. The response may take the form of a long letter or you can write a short covering letter and attach a separate document. The latter may be best if the journal practises masked review and sends revised submissions to reviewers. Either way, remember to quote any reference numbers assigned by the journal.

If, in the course of your revisions, you come across errors or feel inspired to make changes not suggested by the reviewers, you should identify these in the response. In most cases, editors are happy to accept these, since it is easier to make changes at this stage than after typesetting. However, if you have received a conditional acceptance, count your blessings and don't rewrite your paper completely.

Some journals return revised papers to the reviewers. In other cases the editor decides whether the paper is now acceptable. Sometimes journals send papers to a new reviewer, for example for statistical review. Whichever applies, you will get a response to your revised submission. In some cases, you will be asked to make further changes. The same rules apply. Your chances of acceptance rise the more you are prepared to follow the reviewers' comments but, even at this stage, you do not have to do everything they request, so long as you can provide a reasoned explanation for your decision.

If the paper is acceptable to the journal, you will get a final acceptance letter. Keep this in case you want to cite your work elsewhere before it is published, since many journals require a copy of the acceptance letter to prove that a paper is "in press".

What to do if you get an unconditional acceptance

CELEBRATE!

What to do if you think the peer review system has been unfair

Nobody likes having work rejected. So, before you do anything, calm down, set the matter aside for a couple of days and then discuss it with someone experienced in the ways of journals. If your advisor agrees that you have been badly treated, you can consider taking action. In the first place, write to the journal editor and explain your grievance. Provide as many facts and as much documentary evidence as possible but keep a neutral tone and avoid ranting. Unless you know the editor well, always write rather than call in the first instance. In many cases, the editor is the only person you can appeal to, but some journals have an ombudsman who will consider grievances. If the journal is run by a learned society, you could contact the senior officer or appropriate committee.

The Committee on Publication Ethics (COPE) was established to help journal editors resolve difficult cases. It considers anonymised cases submitted by editors and suggests actions. At the moment it does not consider complaints from authors and mostly relates to UK journals, but the accounts of previous cases make interesting reading (see the COPE website at www.publicationethics.co.uk).

What happens after your paper has been accepted

Even if your work is rejected at first, if you are persistent, and realistic about your choice of journals, you should eventually get it accepted somewhere. Once it has been accepted the only thing you need to do is inform the journal if the corresponding author's contact details change, and be patient.

What to do when the proofs arrive

Despite having kept you waiting for several months, most journals expect authors to check and return proofs rapidly. This is why it is important to inform the editor if the corresponding author's contact details change, or if you need to nominate another author for correspondence because the original one is hard to reach. If you do not return the proofs within the deadline, publication may be delayed to the next issue.

Even though you may be short of time, take two copies of the proofs. Give one copy to somebody else to read – two sets of eyes are better than one. Use the second copy for your own marks. Don't mark the original until you have read the entire paper.

Tips for proofreading

- Read the paper several times, each time focusing on different aspects:
  - Read at normal speed to catch the sense and any missing words.
  - Read SLOWLY to check spelling.
  - Read line by line comparing with the typescript to spot errors that have crept in during typesetting (admittedly rarer now that most papers are set from authors' disks, but don't assume they can't happen).
- Concentrate on the ends of words and ends of lines – at normal reading speed these are the places where most mistakes are missed.
- Use a ruler or blank sheet of paper to help you focus on a single line.
- Read words in reverse order or read the paper out loud to slow your reading.
- Read the paper to someone else who checks it against the original typescript. This can be especially helpful for numerical data or large tables.
- Mark your changes clearly, preferably using conventional proofreading marks. These consist of marks within the text and also in the margin.

You can find proofreading marks in *Whittaker's Almanac* and at:
www.m-w.com/mw/table/proofrea.htm
or at
www.ideography.co.uk/proof/marks.html

Queries that arose during copy editing will be marked on the proofs. You can usually mark all changes on the proofs but it may sometimes help to add a covering letter. Remember that the technical editor will have put your paper into the journal's house style. You chose to submit your work to that journal so do not undo these stylistic changes even though they may not be your usual style. If, however, you feel that copy editing has introduced inaccuracies or ambiguities, or the technical editor has misinterpreted your intended meaning, you may correct these, and a polite note explaining your reasons will be helpful.

Electronic proofs

Electronic journals usually ask authors to check both the full text html (the standard web page) and the pdf (the version laid out like a paper journal page for printing). You should check both versions independently as you would for a normal proof. You should also check that the hyperlinks in the html version (for example from reference numbers in the text to the references themselves) are working properly, and that the layout of the pdf is acceptable.

Post-publication peer review

Once your work is published you hope that it will be read and discussed by your peers. This may lead to correspondence in the journal. Electronic journals particularly encourage readers to respond to papers and may post comments on their websites, where, of course, authors can reply. Paper journals often send authors copies of letters that they plan to publish and will publish the authors' responses.

Sometimes, despite peer review and copy editing, mistakes come to light after publication. If this happens you should contact the journal and request a correction. Electronic publishing makes it technically possible to update work after its initial publication. However, not all journals allow this, since they wish to create a permanent record rather than something that changes over time. Some electronic publications, such as the Cochrane Library and BioMed Central, encourage authors to update their work by subsequent submission of a revised and updated article, and to take account of comments made after publication.

How to ensure that your paper is rejected

- Adopt a ponderous and wordy style and try to make everything ambiguous – after all, if readers can understand the stuff, it can't be that clever.
- Insert references to all your previous publications at random, especially if they bear no relation to the current work.
- Ignore the journal's conventions about the structure of abstract and paper.
- If you must follow a structure, ensure that you include some choice results in the methods section and plenty of discussion in the results section.
- Pick a journal at random, or because the title sounds impressive.
- On no account read the instructions to authors.
- Print everything single spaced on an ancient dot-matrix printer.
- If you don't have access to such a printer, make sure the low ink/toner warning light has been flickering for months or, failing that, make illegible photocopies.
- Make sure your pages are not numbered and, if possible, submit them out of order.
- Insert figures and tables into the text as the whim takes you.
- Choose an obscure style for references (and definitely not that of your chosen journal).
- Remember not to check your references and ensure that several are incomplete.
- Make sure that you exceed the maximum length by at least 1000 words and two tables.
- If you have trouble with this, paste paragraphs from your supervisor's previous publications into your introduction and discussion.
- Try to include some figures in a format the journal cannot print, such as colour photographs.
- Submit the manuscript without a covering letter.
- If you must write a letter, leave out vital contact details for the corresponding author.
- Alternatively, enclose a handwritten note addressed to an editor who died several years ago.

Surviving peer review of conference abstracts

Getting an abstract accepted is the key to presenting your findings at a conference. Unlike journals, most meeting organisers set a strict deadline for submitting abstracts and usually provide detailed instructions about their length and format, even the font (typeface and size) to use.

In most cases, review involves a simple accept/reject decision and you will not get a chance to revise your abstract, so it is particularly important to pay attention to detail and follow the instructions provided. In most cases abstracts are submitted as "camera-ready", that is they will appear exactly as they are submitted. Electronic submission is increasingly common (and a lot easier than messing about with typewriters and correction fluid) but, because of time constraints, most abstracts are still accepted as submitted.

Follow the instructions provided, which often suggest a structure for the abstract and the headings you should use (for example: Objective, Methods, Results, Discussion). If the organisers require a particular structure, you should follow it precisely. If no structure is specified consider whether headings would be helpful. Using headings makes abstracts easier to read but it also makes them longer. Ignore the word/ space limits at your peril!

In most cases, abstracts should not contain tables or references.

If results are not available by the submission deadline, be realistic about submitting an abstract promising findings. If you are really sure that you will have data in time for the conference, prepare an abstract making the rationale for your research as enticing as possible and concentrate on explaining the methods clearly. In some cases, the methods themselves may form the basis for the submission (for example, if you've developed a new rating scale).

If you need co-authors' or supervisor's agreement or permission before you submit, take this into account and give them plenty of time to review the abstract before the submission deadline.

Make the reviewers' job as easy as possible. Explain all abbreviations and make them as meaningful as possible (for example, instead of referring to treatment groups 1 and 2, consider using A for active and P for placebo or C for control).

How to ensure that you never present your work at a conference

- Pick the conference solely by the exotic destination.
- Miss the abstract deadline by several weeks.
- Make sure your abstract exceeds the maximum length.
- Try to go over all four borders of the abstract template.
- Include tables or figures in your abstract to pad it out.
- Prepare your abstract on your aunt's ancient typewriter with an equally antique ribbon.
- Better still, ask your aunt to type it for you from an illegible hand-written copy to ensure plenty of spelling mistakes.
- Omit vital details of your methods or results (preferably both).
- Omit results altogether and write "findings will be presented".
- Submit your abstract by fax or email if this is expressly forbidden.
- Submit the wrong abstract (preferably one that you have presented several times before on a totally different subject).

Surviving peer review of grant proposals

Grant proposals involve translating your study protocol into a request for funding from one or more institutions. The same general rules for submission apply as for journals but, like conference abstracts, there may be a strict deadline for submission.

First:

- make sure the charity or grant giving body you choose is the right one by checking that it supports work in your field;
- read the instructions;
- stick to timelines, format, and length;
- invite informal peer review from knowledgeable outsiders.

To increase your chances of getting funded, you need to:

- make the case that there is a need for your particular study or intended course of action;
- convince reviewers that you are equipped to carry out the task.

Is the research needed?

The most convincing grant proposals put the need for the proposed study into the context of current knowledge of the subject. The best way to do this is to use the findings of one or more systematic reviews of the broad topic area. If relevant Cochrane reviews are available, this will make your life easier, as these usually finish with an exhortation to further research (check the Cochrane Library at www.cochrane.co.uk). More and more commissioning and funding bodies are turning to the results of systematic reviews to identify gaps in knowledge.

If a systematic review of the topic area is not available, you should carry out a thorough review of the evidence yourself. You can do this by searching electronic databases such as Medline and Embase for published articles, and the *meta*Register of Controlled Trials (www.controlled-trials.com) for planned or ongoing research.

Are you the right people to do the work?

A convincing demonstration on paper of the need for your study is the first crucial ingredient for a successful application, but are you (or is your team) up to the job of filling the gap in knowledge that you have identified? You must convince reviewers that you are. You should do this by writing as clearly and exhaustively as possible. The more time you spend on your proposal and the better quality it is, the more chance you will have of convincing funding bodies to put their faith (and their cash) in you. When you are calculating the resources required, be as clear as the format allows you. If you believe your explanation is constrained by the format requested you can add a separate sheet. Bear in mind that larger charities or bodies may have reviewers specifically assessing the financial side of the proposal, so they should be able to make sense of it without full reference to the rest of the protocol.

Last, but not least, take care in producing or updating your curriculum vitae (resumé or CV), which almost all charities or funding bodies require with your application. This will be scrutinised as carefully as, and in some cases more carefully than, the proposal itself. You may consider editing your CV to highlight a particular expertise that matches the skills required for the study.

5: Professional peer review

Professional appraisal systems, especially those for nurses, are often referred to as peer review. They may involve assessment by peers (that is, colleagues at the same level) and by bosses and supervisors or even junior colleagues. Unlike the processes used to review submissions to journals, conferences, or funding bodies, these assessments take place face to face. The aim of the process is to review performance and identify both strengths and problems. For many people, receiving or delivering such feedback can be embarrassing or uncomfortable. This chapter suggests techniques for making professional peer review a positive experience for everyone.

The guidelines are written from the point of view of people doing the appraisal, because they have a more active part in making the meeting productive. However, the information will be relevant to those who are being appraised since, if you are on the receiving end of badly handled peer review, your only hope of improving the situation is to give good feedback to the appraisers to make them understand their own limitations.

Principles of peer reviewing another person's performance

Review the performance, not the person. Personal criticisms not only injure the individual and damage relationships, but are unproductive and sometimes even counterproductive. Telling someone that they are stupid or lazy gives no indication about how you would like them to improve, and only tells the appraisee that you don't like them.

Be specific. Focus on specific behaviours. Vagueness does not make criticism gentler and, like personal attacks, may leave the appraisee bewildered as to what they have done wrong. Avoid generalisations and terms like "always"; they will only make the other person defensive. If you say, "You are always late for work", the appraisee is likely to counter with examples of days when he or she was on time. The professional peer review then descends into an argument, which helps nobody. It is better to say, "You were late for work last Wednesday and both the previous Mondays". This is far less likely to elicit a defensive reaction and more likely to bring forth an explanation or apology.

Don't make assumptions. State the facts, as you understand them, then let the other person tell their story. Avoid adding your own interpretation or guessing others' motives. Remember that you may be wrong, or misinformed. Be particularly wary of passing on concerns or information reported to you by others. If you need to do this, always make this clear. Where possible, report only facts you are sure of. For example, do not say, "You are unhelpful to junior colleagues", if you have not witnessed this; say instead, "Your junior colleagues have approached me saying that they would like more help." Avoiding second-hand criticism will obviate arguments and give the other person a chance to tell their side of the story.

Explain the consequences of the appraisee's actions. Most people do not set out to be a nuisance and may honestly believe that their way of doing something is best. It is not sufficient to expect someone to do something "because I told you to". Treat the other person with respect and like an adult, and give reasons why you would like their behaviour to change. For example, "When you are late, the nurses on the night shift have to stay late and they often miss the bus back to the hostel."

Do your homework. Gather specific examples and, if necessary, corroborate your evidence. If done sensitively and routinely, this need not appear like a witch-hunt. Questionnaires to colleagues can be part of the process, and are especially useful when reviewing the work of somebody who spends time in several departments or who works for different managers. So called "360-degree review" involves collecting information not only from a person's managers and peers, but also from their subordinates and junior colleagues. Such information is usually anonymised and the people giving the feedback should be given guidance about the process and what is expected of them.

Apologise if you discover you were wrong. If you have received incorrect information, made a wrong assumption, or find that an event was somebody else's fault, do not hesitate to apologise, then move on to another topic.

Agree specific actions for improvement. The more specific your recommendations, the easier they will be to understand, and the more likely everyone is to agree whether they have been followed or not. If you feel you must impose a sanction, for example requiring supervision for certain procedures, make sure that you agree a timescale and agree to review progress at the end of this.

Set realistic targets. Be objective and think about the behaviour that you are willing to accept from other people. Do not set stricter measures than this for the person who has disappointed you. Unfair sanctions or anything that appears vindictive or punitive will only be demotivating.

Don't be overprescriptive. Although you should clearly describe the outcome you want, it is usually best to leave the other person to decide how this can be achieved. However, be prepared to give more detail or to answer questions if the appraisee requests this.

Use open questions to elicit information. Open questions cannot be answered with yes or no, so they are useful for obtaining information. They force the other person to use their own words rather than echoing yours. Even if you think that you know the reason for something, it is better to let the appraisee explain. So ask, "Why were you late on Tuesday?" rather than saying "On Tuesday mornings you take your son to the nursery, don't you?" Some famous lines by Kipling summarise the techniques of open questioning:

> *I had my six good serving men, they taught me all I knew,*
> *Their names were, how and why and what,*
> *and when and where and who.*

Give the appraisee a chance to speak. Do not be afraid of silences – although they can feel uncomfortable. Avoid the temptation of filling in for the other person. State your facts, ask open questions, then wait for the answer.

Use techniques of active listening. Give the person your full attention, encourage them by nodding and saying things like, "Yes" and "Go on". Do not look at your watch or diary and try not to make notes all the time. Make occasional eye contact but avoid fixing the appraisee with an inquisitorial stare.

Use closed questions to summarise or gain agreement. Closed questions can be answered with yes or no. Although unhelpful when you are trying to understand another person's story, they can be useful at the end of a discussion to confirm agreement or understanding.

Remember to praise as well as criticise. Routinely praising one behaviour before you criticise another can appear formulaic and insincere. Instead, remember to put negative feedback in the context of overall performance. Don't be embarrassed to praise good performance and, like criticism, make this as specific as possible and explain why it had good consequences. If someone's overall performance is good, make this very clear, both before and after you discuss their occasional lapses or areas for improvement. If someone has done something you consider to be out of character, it may be helpful to express your concern or disappointment. For example, "You have been so helpful to X since she joined the unit last month, that I was surprised when she told me that you refused to help her with ... last week."

Don't spring surprises. An annual or quarterly professional peer review gives a chance to review a person's work fully and provides time for discussion, but it should not be used as an excuse to limit feedback to these scheduled, formal sessions. It is far better to provide feedback as soon as something has occurred. Do not store things up for the appraisal – memories will have faded, facts become obscured and the appraisee is likely to feel "got at". People are more likely to get upset if criticism comes as a shock to them. When providing immediate feedback, use the same principles of addressing the behaviour, not the person, and being as specific as possible. Avoid criticising somebody in public, especially in front of colleagues.

Style matters

How you say something is often as important as what you say, and body language plays a large part in this. If you are conducting an appraisal discussion try to:

- *Be punctual.* Keeping the other person waiting suggests you do not take the process seriously or are playing power games to show how important you are.
- *Be prepared.* Gather your facts well in advance and think about what you are going to say; when the appraisee arrives try to greet the person with a clear desk, the relevant papers ready and your previous piece of work completed.
- *Be attentive.* Give the appraisee your full attention. Avoid fidgeting with papers or other displacement activity, looking at your watch, or doing anything else during the meeting except for speaking and listening. Switch off your mobile phone and, if possible, divert your telephone.

A few more hints

Address issues in order of importance. Tackle the big things first, to ensure they get sufficient time. The appraisee usually knows his or her own shortcomings or the problems you will want to address and will not concentrate properly on other aspects until the major ones have been addressed.

Focus on solutions. You are not conducting the appraisal to apportion blame or elicit an apology. Aim to review past performance with a view to what can be learned, and perhaps improved, in the future. Avoid dwelling on problems that arose in truly exceptional circumstances.

Don't be afraid to tell the other person how you felt. Telling someone that you felt hurt, let down or embarrassed by their behaviour is more powerful than resorting to personal abuse. It is also indisputable – you are simply reporting your own feelings.

Peer review often involves a panel of people. If you are a member of such a panel, try to observe these principles yourself and also take responsibility for making sure that other panel members do the same. If someone starts to make vague allegations, ask them to be more specific. If they make a personal attack, try to bring them back to focus on particular behaviour, the problems it can cause, and solutions for the future.

Being on the receiving end

If you are on the receiving end of badly handled professional peer review, try not to get upset. Instead, calmly ask for clarification, examples, and solutions. Avoid becoming defensive if somebody makes generalisations such as "You always do this ...". Equally, avoid exaggerations, such as "I never do that". Prepare your facts (if necessary check dates and times and bring evidence if you think something will be disputed). Apologise for your mistakes or times when your performance was below standard – we are only human and should not be expected to be perfect. Listen to the feedback. It is very easy to hear only the negative parts and forget the positive. If you feel able, you may wish to ask for a follow-up meeting to give your appraiser feedback on how he or she handled your appraisal. In this case, it would be wise to consult your human resources department for advice. And remember, one day you are likely to be on the other side of the table, so use any bad experiences to learn how to do professional peer review better yourself.

6: Informal peer review

Have you ever asked a colleague to read through something that you have written, then seethed over his or her comments? Have you ever vowed never to show anything to that exasperating nit-picker again? If so, you have not mastered the art of informal peer review. Colleagues' comments can be helpful, and few set out deliberately to injure your feelings, so where do we go wrong? This chapter sets out some principles about requesting feedback on anything you write and on giving helpful reviews to colleagues.

Asking for feedback

Most people don't give the request much thought, and therefore don't give the reviewer much help. How often have you heard someone say "Will you look over this for me, please?" and leave it at that? This is asking for trouble. You will avoid much frustration if you select reviewers for specific skills and give them clear directions. In a work's early stages you might ask someone to comment on the overall structure, whether the arguments flow logically, and whether you have omitted anything vital. However, at this stage, you do not want anyone to polish the punctuation or tell you that the references need reformatting. Make this absolutely clear: tell the reviewer what you want them to do and what you don't want them to do – and give them a deadline. Even if the person is important (your boss, for example), negotiating a deadline is essential. Leaving it open and hoping that reviewers are telepathic will only lead to embarrassment when you have to chase them for comments that you had hoped would have been provided weeks ago.

Ask different people to bring their particular skill to reviewing a paper.

The following might be helpful:

- an expert in the field to check scientific content and advise on references;
- a statistician to check statistical methods and presentation of results;
- a typical reader of the target journal, especially if you are writing for an audience different from yourself (for example, a specialist writing for generalists);
- a naïve reader (someone who does not have your specialist training but will spot flaws in the logic);
- someone who is good at grammar and spelling;
- a native speaker, if you are not writing in your mother tongue.

When you are finalising a piece of work, call on a reviewer who is good at "micro-editing": someone who will spot spelling mistakes and is good at grammar and punctuation. You don't want someone to tell you to rewrite the piece or radically change its structure if a deadline is looming. Your micro-editor doesn't have to be an expert in the subject; an eye for detail is more important at this stage.

If you ask a statistician to review a paper, you will be doing them a favour if you explain that somebody else is checking the grammar and that you expect the statistician to focus on the statistical methods section and check that the results are displayed sensibly. This is not to imply that statisticians are illiterate, but they are usually busy so use their talents where they are most needed: on the statistics. Ideally, you should have involved statisticians at an early stage in the design of the study. Do not expect them to breathe life into a hopelessly flawed study by statistical wizardry when you come to write it up. The same goes for health economists.

After you have given your reviewers clear instructions and agreed a deadline, leave them in peace. Don't hover while they are reading. Even if you want an instant response on an abstract, go away and have a cup of coffee to give them a chance to read the whole thing through without interruptions.

Finally, don't forget to thank all reviewers and, where appropriate, formally acknowledge their input in the work. Remember to give them a reprint or final copy.

Giving feedback

If you are given clear instructions (see above) giving feedback is easy. If someone simply asks you to read and review something, get more details before you begin.

> **Points to ask before reviewing:**
> - What kind of review is expected?
> - What stage is the work at (1st draft or pre-final)?
> - Who is it written for?
> - Where will it be published/presented?
> - Who else has reviewed/will review it?
> - What form should comments take (paper, electronic, verbal)?
> - What is the deadline?

Always consider the other person's feelings when you make comments. Remember that a paper or report may be the final phase of several years' work. However bad you think it is, find something to praise. If your comments are relatively minor, make sure you emphasise this and say how good other aspects are. If you suggest major changes, it is best to talk them through with the author, either in person or over the telephone.

Be specific. Vagueness is not kindness and instructions to "Rewrite this section" or "Pay attention to grammar" are not helpful. If you discover a repeated problem, highlight this tactfully, don't become exasperated. Coach the person so that they learn from the experience of your review and you stay friends. Copying a page from a style guide or writing book can be helpful to explain grammatical mistakes (the older edition of Fowler's *Modern English Usage* provides helpful explanations for confusion over "that" and "which", for example). If you really like somebody but find their writing style turgid, buy them a copy of *Strunk & White* (see the Further Reading section for details).

The style of a review is as important as its content. Avoid sarcasm, patronising remarks and anything that sounds like a school report. Use blue or green ink rather than red. (This sounds trivial but it makes a difference; reserve red ink for your own work or thick-skinned authors.)

Thank the person for asking you to review their work. After all, it is a sign that they respect your views (unless you happen to be their boss).

How not to do informal review

- Make sure you miss the deadline and submit your review late.
- Despite missing the deadline, set aside time when you are in a rush, preferably at the end of a bad day, with a migraine brewing or after a row with your boss.
- Phrase all your remarks as questions, preferably sarcastic ones. (Use the word "surely" as much as possible, for example *"Surely not"*.)
- Insert exclamation marks at the end of each paragraph.
- If you have few comments, make sure you counteract this with a cover note telling the writer that this is a lousy piece of work.
- Expect the writer to be telepathic:

  - If you can't manage a full question, simply scrawl large question marks in the margin and give the writer no indication of what you are concerned about.
  - Demand further references, but don't provide any clues to identify them.
  - Ensure your writing is illegible.

- Make sure you are unfamiliar with the intended journal's requirements and insist on changes that contravene these.
- Change UK to US spelling (or vice versa) regardless of the intended journal's style or, even better, inconsistently.
- Make your comments as ambiguous as possible.
- Intersperse comments with notes to yourself, doodles, shopping lists, etc.
- Phrase your corrections with as much emotion as possible.
- Wherever possible add a personal attack on the intelligence of the writer.
- Be arrogant and claim expertise you do not have.
- Use thick red marker pen and triple underlining (especially on the personal attacks).
- Sound increasingly exasperated as you progress through the manuscript.
- Point out minor changes to punctuation but later suggest that the entire section should be deleted or rewritten.
- Point out every tiny typo and punctuation problem, especially if you've been asked to comment only on the structure of a very early draft.
- Retype large sections with no indication of where you have made changes (and only provide this as hard copy to ensure the writer has to retype as much as possible).
- Suggest a radical rethink of structure and key messages on the fifth draft (having okayed the previous four).
- Act on the basis of ignorance – save your most forceful criticisms for sections dealing with topics in which you have the least knowledge.
- Hold your prejudices to the fore.

Getting feedback from potential readers

If you are writing for people who do not share your background or training, you should seek feedback from potential readers. This applies if you are writing for another professional group or another specialty, but especially if you are writing for patients or carers. The closer your audience resembles you, the easier it will be to write for them. Writing for lay people is a particular skill, outside the scope of this book (see the Further Reading section for more help). Seeking comments from patients also poses special problems, but is an essential step in producing material that is helpful to them.

Patients or carers may be surprised if a healthcare professional asks for their views on a document. You should therefore explain why you are asking them to review something and exactly what you want them to do. Patients may be embarrassed to refuse a request from a doctor or nurse, so you should give them time to consider their decision and avoid making your request in front of other people. If possible, give them an opportunity to read the piece first and then let you know if they are prepared to comment on it.

As with all reviewers, be specific. Explain exactly what you want. Verbal feedback may be easier to provide than written (not everybody has a computer) and less daunting, especially if you listen attentively and encourage the reviewer. Remember that it can be very intimidating to be the lone patient or layperson in a room of healthcare professionals, so try to invite more than one and give them a chance to discuss their views together (and/or with you) before the meeting. People feel more confident if they know that others share their views, and there is safety in numbers. Offer to meet patients' expenses to attend meetings.

As with all other reviewers, thank them for their input, acknowledge them wherever possible, and make sure they see the final version.

Other situations where informal peer review can be used

You can use informal peer review to improve anything you have written, from a letter to a book. If you "train" your reviewers well, understand their expertise, and give clear instructions the process should be painless for both parties. Over time, you will build a pool of trusted advisors and, if all goes well, you will benefit from their input. However, you may also discover that some people will never understand the principles of peer review. Avoid colleagues who see a review as an opportunity to score points, be spiteful, or progress their own careers at the expense of yours. Develop a thick skin for people whose opinions you value but who have not learned the art of constructive criticism – or buy them a copy of this book.

Further reading

Books

Writing style

Fowler HW. *A dictionary of modern English usage, 2nd ed.* Oxford: Oxford University Press, 1965. (The completely revised edition is a much less helpful and authoritative guide.)
Strunk WJ, White EB. *The elements of style, 3rd ed.* Needham Heights, Massachusetts: Allyn & Bacon, 1979. (Also available at http://www.columbia.edu/acis/bartleby)

Scientific style

Council of Biology Editors. *Scientific style and format: The CBE manual for authors, editors, and publishers, 6th ed.* Cambridge: Cambridge University Press, 1994.

Medical writing and publishing

Albert T. *A-Z of medical writing.* London: BMJ Books, 2000.
Albert T. *Winning the publications game.* Abingdon, Oxon: Radcliffe Medical Press, 1997.
Fraser J. *How to publish in biomedicine: 500 tips for success.* Abingdon, Oxon: Radcliffe Medical Press, 1997.
Goodman NW, Edwards MB. *Medical writing a prescription for clarity, 2nd ed.* Cambridge: Cambridge University Press, 1997.
Hall GM (ed). *How to write a paper, 2nd ed.* London: BMJ Books, 1998.
Lang TA, Secic M. *How to report statistics in medicine: annotated guidelines for authors, editors, and reviewers.* Philadelphia: American College of Physicians, 1997.

Peer review

Godlee F, Jefferson T (eds). *Peer review in health sciences.* London: BMJ Books, 1999.
Jones AH, McLellan F (eds). *Ethical issues in biomedical publication.* Baltimore, Maryland: Johns Hopkins University Press, 2000.
Lock S. *A difficult balance: editorial peer review in medicine.* London: BMJ Books, 1991.

Methodological review

Altman D. *Statistics with confidence, 2nd ed.* London: BMJ Books, 2000.
Egger M, Davey-Smith G, Altman D. *Systematic reviews in health care.* London: BMJ Books, 2001.
Greenhalgh T. *How to read a paper.* London: BMJ Books, 1997.
Jadad A. *Randomised controlled trials.* London: BMJ Books, 1998.
Sackett DL, Haynes RB, Guyatt GH, Tugwell P. *Clinical epidemiology, a basic science for clinical medicine 2nd ed.* Baltimore: Lippincott, Williams & Wilkins, 1991.

Journal articles

Methodological review

Begg C, Cho M, Eastwood S *et al.* Improving the quality of reporting of randomized controlled trials. The CONSORT statement. *JAMA* 1996;**276**: 637–9.
Drummond MF, Jefferson TO *et al.* Guidelines for authors and peer-reviewers of economic submissions to the British Medical Journal. *BMJ* 1996;**313**:275–83.
Ketchum P. Checklists for excellence. *Can Family Physician* 1998;**44**:2193–201.
Moher D, Shulz KF, Altman DG. The CONSORT statement: revised recommendations for improving the quality of parallel-group randomised trials. *Lancet* 2001;**357**:1191–4. (Also available on www.consort-statement.org)
Moher D, Cook DJ, Eastwood S *et al.* Improving the quality of reports of meta-analyses of randomised controlled trials: the QUOROM statement. Quality of Reporting of Meta-analyses. *Lancet* 1999; **354**:1896–900.

Professional peer review

Maguire D. Ten Commandments of peer review. *Neonatal Network* 1998;**17**:63–7.
Micheli AJ, Modest S. Peer review. *Nurs Clinics N Amer* 1995;**30**:197–210.

Useful websites

Cochrane collaboration: www.cochrane.org
CONSORT statement: www.consort-statement.org
Commission on Publication Ethics (COPE): www.publicationethics.org uk
Council of Science Editors (CSE): www.CouncilScienceEditors.org
Glossary of printing and typography: http://home.vicnet.net.au/~typo/glossary/index.htm
Instructions for authors (helpful even if you are not submitting to these journals): www.bmj.com and www.thelancet.com
International Committee of Medical Journal Editors (ICMJE) Uniform requirements for submission to biomedical journals: www.icmje.org
Medline (PubMed) database: www.pubmed.org
Newcastle/Ottawa scale for assessing the quality of non-randomised studies: www.lri.ca/programs/ceu/oxford.htm
Proofreading marks: www.ideography.co.uk/proof/marks.html and www.m-w.com/mw/table/proofrea.htm
World Association of Medical Editors (WAME): www.wame.org

Methodological review checklists

General questions

- Why was the study done?
- Have the authors adequately reviewed existing research?
- Was there a clearly defined question?
- What study design was used?
- Was the design right for the question? (See below.)
- Was the study ethical?
- Are the conclusions justified?

Matching the question to the study design

Question	Study design
Does the treatment work?	RCT or systematic review of RCTs
How good is this diagnostic test?	Prospective cohort study
Is screening effective?	RCT
What causes this disease?	Prospective cohort study/ case control study
What is the prognosis?	Prospective cohort study
What do people think?	Cross sectional survey/ cohort survey (over time)

Systematic reviews and meta-analyses

- Did the authors search adequately and without bias for all relevant studies?
- Did they use appropriate criteria to decide which studies to include in the review (based on study design, interventions, outcome measures, populations, sample size)?
- Was selection and methodological assessment of studies done in a reproducible and unbiased way (for example, by

two independent assessors, blinded to the results of the studies)?

- Were the studies comparable on clinical grounds (interventions, outcomes, population)?
- If the authors combined the studies for statistical analysis, were the right statistical methods used (fixed effects or random effects model)?
- Did the authors perform sensitivity analyses to see whether excluding or including different studies, or performing alternative statistical tests, made a difference to the results?
- Is the difference between the groups statistically significant? If so, is it clinically significant?
- Can you tell from the report how many people would need to be treated with the new treatment rather than the old to achieve one additional positive outcome (number needed to treat) or to cause one additional adverse effect (number needed to harm)?

Randomised controlled trials (RCTs)

- Were the outcomes clinically important (for example, survival or mobility rather than results of blood tests or x rays)?
- Was a power calculation performed to determine the sample size needed to detect a clinically important difference?
- Was allocation to treatments randomised?
- Was the method of randomisation adequately described?
- Was the allocation of patients to the different arms of the trial arranged so that no one could predict which treatment the patient would receive (allocation concealment, using, for example, opaque envelopes or calls to a randomisation service)?
- Except for the intervention being tested, were the groups treated exactly the same?
- Was compliance to treatment (adherence) assessed?
- Were the outcomes assessed by people who were unaware of which treatment the patient had received (blinded outcome assessment)?
- Were all patients properly accounted for (for example, people who were excluded before or after randomisation, withdrew from treatment, did not comply, or could not be followed up)?

- Was follow-up adequate (more than 85%)?
- Were patients analysed in the groups they were randomised to (intention to treat analysis)?
- Is the difference between the groups statistically significant? If so, is it clinically significant? If not statistically significant, was the study large enough to detect a clinically significant difference?
- Can you tell from the report how many people need to be treated with the new treatment rather than the old to achieve one additional positive outcome (number needed to treat) or to cause one additional adverse effect (number needed to harm)?

Studies of prognosis

- Did the authors gather an inception cohort (patients identified at an early, uniform, and well-defined point in the course of the disease)?
- Was referral into the study unbiased and clearly described?
- Was complete follow up achieved?
- Were outcome criteria objective, reproducible, and accurate, and were they assessed blind?
- Did the authors adjust for extraneous prognostic factors?

Studies evaluating diagnostic tests

- Was the new test compared with the current gold standard test?
- Were both gold standard and new tests performed on all participants?
- Do the authors adequately describe the setting for the study (for example, primary care or tertiary care) and the criteria for deciding which patients to include?
- Did the sample include a full range of people with mild and severe, treated and untreated disease, as well as people with other disorders that fall within the differential diagnosis?
- Do the authors describe the new test in sufficient detail to allow others to replicate it?
- Does the study assess whether the test is reproducible (precision) and whether different observers agree on interpretation (observer variation)?

- Was the term "normal" defined sensibly?
- Does the study assess whether the patients were really better off as a result of having the test (utility)?

Studies of causation

- Did the authors use the best possible study design (prospective cohort study, or case control study for rare diseases)?
- Were the opportunities for and the determination of exposure free from bias?
- Is the relative risk/odds ratio significantly greater than 1? If so, is the increased risk clinically significant? If not statistically significant, was the study large enough to detect a clinically significant difference?

Cohort studies

- Is it clear how the cohort was recruited?
- Did the authors consider factors that might influence the type of people included in the cohort (for example, reasons why more severely ill people might have been excluded)?
- If the study used hard endpoints such as death, were all events identified?
- If the study used "softer" endpoints, were all measurement tools (such as questionnaires) properly validated?
- Were severity of disease and presence of other diseases taken into account in the analysis?

Case control studies

- Does the study adequately describe how cases were defined?
- Were the controls appropriate?
- Did the controls match the cases in every necessary way except the disease/risk factor under study?
- Were data collected in the same way for cases and controls?
- Were measurements free from bias?
- Do the authors take account of all possible sources of confounding?

Surveys

- Are the aims clearly stated?
- Was the selection of subjects (sampling) unbiased and adequately described?
- Was the questionnaire validated in terms of intra- and inter-rater reliability?
- Does the questionnaire measure the things that matter?
- Was the sample size justified?
- Was the response rate adequate?
- Did the authors look for important differences between responders and non-responders?

Qualitative studies

- Did the authors adequately describe the setting and the method of sampling?
- Were attempts made to minimise subjectivity during data collection?
- Did the authors take steps to maximise the reliability of the data (for example, repeated data collection by a second independent researcher)?
- Did the authors separate the results from their interpretation?

Economic analyses

- Were the alternative healthcare programmes adequately described?
- Has their effectiveness been assessed in RCTs? If not, do the authors clearly identify the sources of their effectiveness estimates?
- Were all important costs and effects identified?
- Did the study use credible measures of these costs and effects?
- Were the analyses appropriate?

The checklists have been adapted from Sackett D, Haynes B, Tugwell P, Guyatt G. *Clinical Epidemiology – A Basic Science for Clinical Medicine, 2nd edn* with permission from Lippincott, Williams & Wilkins.

Glossary

(Entries referring to other items in the glossary are shown in *italics*.)

Authors' editor A professional writer/editor usually employed by the authors' institution to help prepare publications and grant applications. More common in the US than in Europe.

Blinding/blinded review The process of removing the authors' details from a paper before it is sent to reviewers in an attempt to mask the authors' identity. Also called *masking*.

CONSORT A set of guidelines for reporting the results of randomised controlled trials (see Further reading for more details).

Content expert Someone working in the relevant scientific or medical field, as distinct from a methodology expert or statistician.

Copy editor Alternative name for a *technical editor*.

Corresponding author The author whose full contact details appear on a publication and who is the point of contact with the journal for handling reviewers' comments, proofs, etc.

Editor The Editor (with a capital "E") of a journal (sometimes called the Editor-in-Chief) is the person in overall charge, who makes final decisions about acceptance, policy, etc. Sometimes there will be an Academic Editor, responsible for content, and a Managing Editor responsible for running the journal. Larger journals may employ several editors who handle papers and also *technical editors* (or *subeditors*).

Embase Commercial database of medical references maintained by Excerpta Medica, who charge for its use. Contains a wider range of journals than *Medline*.

Galley proofs   Proofs set in a single column before being made up into pages (increasingly rare since the introduction of computer typesetting and largely replaced by *page proofs*).

House style   Style imposed by a journal on anything to be published. It will include things such as the typeface of headings, the format of references, the type of abstract used, conventions for abbreviations, etc.

HTML   HyperText Mark-up Language: a computer code used to create electronic journals and web pages.

ICMJE   International Committee of Medical Journal Editors (also called the Vancouver Group) – a group of journal editors who prepared the Uniform Requirements for Submissions to Biomedical Journals and who issue occasional statements about aspects of publication such as authorship and conflicts of interest.

Medline   Electronic database of abstracts of articles from biomedical journals (with a strong bias towards those in English) produced by the *National Library of Medicine*. Available free at: www.ncbi.nlm.nih.gov/PubMed

MeSH headings   Medical Subject Headings – system of medical terms used by the *National Library of Medicine* and often adopted for journal keywords.

Micro-editing   Making changes to grammar, spelling, etc. without altering the overall structure of a piece of writing.

National Library of Medicine   US government-funded library providing services such as *Medline*.

Page proofs   Proofs in the form that the final pages will appear (cf *galley proofs*).

Pay journal   A journal that charges a fee for publication, either in the form of a page charge or a requirement to buy a certain number of reprints.

PDF files   Portable Document Format: electronic files designed to be printed rather than read directly from a website.

Manuscript   Strictly speaking, a handwritten document, but often used to refer to any unpublished submission. More correctly these are referred to as *typescripts*.

Masking   The process of removing the authors' details from a paper before it is sent to reviewers, and of removing the reviewers' identities from any comments sent to authors. The opposite of *open review*. Sometimes called *blinding*.

Open review   Peer review in which the author knows the identity of the reviewer and vice versa.

Referee   Name sometimes given to *reviewers* who are asked to advise a journal on whether a submission should be accepted.

Reviewer   Somebody who assesses work for scientific content and presentation and offers opinions about the originality, usefulness, ethical and methodological soundness of the study and the accuracy and clarity of the reporting.

Technical editor   Somebody who puts accepted papers into the journal's house style, edits the language and checks for completeness and consistency (also called a *subeditor or copy-editor*).

Typescript   An unpublished submission, often (pedants would say incorrectly) called a *manuscript*.

Index

Page numbers in *italic* refer to tables or boxed material.